COVID-19

RUMOR

AND

REALITY

Covid-19 Rumor Surpasses The Reality   Assigning A Complex Pandemic

Kishore Baran Nath

TABLE OF CONTENTS

PROLOGUE

The Novel Coronavirus or Covid-19, wearing a huge crown is dominating the world. The world was almost traumatized by its heinous kingship. The virus has become the only villain in the horror movie. Though his power seems to decline while we are talking about him after nine months of his emergence, scare is still everywhere. All should have pain for the gloomy reality that the disease has actually had. But who ought to admire what should not have been done with us? We see, the selfish took full advantage of the pandemic, spread panic, involved in corruption for business and overall, has made it a drama of panic.

Still, constant messages are telling us that he is not to stop right now and any negligence might cause big havoc. Finding no other alternatives to save the economy, lockdown has been relaxed or some countries are preparing for further lockdown. The world is recommended to maintain social distance, wear a mask, wash hands and do everything possible because any time, he may swoop down again too badly. We still see that hundreds or thousands of people are dying every day and many are being infected. It is said that People shall have to look forward to the coronavirus vaccine to prevent the killer disease.

It emerged in December of 2019 in Wuhan of China, spread over the whole world and has grasped the throats of millions of people till now. He has gone on devastating dance making the world restless in fear, paralyzed in lockdown. Now the world is seeing the light of hope for the corona vaccine invention.

While the world is still in fear and striving for a vaccine, I am trying to look into the reality of coronavirus.

I am going to show you a picture of the rumor and reality of that giant virus or the pandemic. By the end of this journey you will see how absurd and unwise the lockdown was, how illogical and baseless the scare was in which we are still living. You will find no other way than rethinking on every element of the Covid Pandemic. You will find if the crisis was lotted to the world or the world destined itself to that unlimited crisis.

You will find if it was the only way that we have been shown to face a pandemic like Covid, or there are good alternatives to logically fight and live in the world. You will also find the pandemics or the definition of pandemics questionable with a bit of absorption.

I believe a good thinker will never say that that kind of lockdown and horrific presentation of the disease has or should have a reasonable ground. A rational being will never be able to support that whole paralysis by lockdown if he travels through the data and statistics to find out a way.

I will show you a vivid picture of coronavirus pandemic which is largely different from that you have heard and experienced so far. I will try to make a good exposure of the pandemic entitling the factor "Rumor and Reality". You will see how the pandemic has been made a drama of scare by the corrupted and selfish where the reality of the disease has been too much exaggerated by panicking the world with unjustified scare.

Most probably, you will find that the world is under a psychological game in the name of Novel Coronavirus.

A virus or say, coronavirus disease has its natural havoc. But we should try to justify if the virus is as dreadful as is said. I think, going inside the writings, you might ask yourselves a question "Is Covid-19 a scandal to befool the world or is it real?" You might ask how much it is real and how much it is crowned with rumor. You might ask if that unjustified scare was uncontrollable or it was intentional and awkward.

I should not like to be a parrot uttering the given words without a bit of thinking and I think, you will like a rational being amidst you. I hope you will find answers to all of your questions by the end of this pandemic journey -- a journey of data and statistics coupled with reasoning and applying common sense. And no big Science is required for you to understand what I am going to talk about.

CHAPTER 1

Pandemic Tragedy

In the middle of covid-19 pandemic, many absurd happenings turn some conscious people's eyes to the past pandemics of the world. Travelling through the past memories, eyes halt at the most recent pandemic and suspect links between pandemics. Most of us may not have known that we had a pandemic stigma, the saddest and totally unbelievable. Swine flu, the so called pandemic only for business, only to plunder money by the token of service for mankind!

Ten years back in 2009, a fully intentional scare was spread in the name of Swine flu. As infection by influenza was rising in Mexico in February of the year, the sample of the virus was sent to the United States and Canada. Instantly the scientists of those countries declared that the virus was too aggressive. The panel specialists of the World Health Organization (WHO) sharply predicted that one third of the world population might have got infected by the virus and out of them, millions would have died. Educational institutes, flights were closed following a rapid lockdown. As a consequence, the Government of Mexico had to accept a big loss of economy -- $ 2.25 billion. Patients got admitted to hospitals ten times as much as they had capacity. Not a mere epidemic, the authorities proclaimed it a pandemic. Worldwide scare made its way to the pinnacle. Professor Anderson, Health advisor of British Government said that the only way to get safe from the disease is to take "Tamiflu fill". Otherwise, people will die.

$ 10 billion worth of Fill and Vaccine had gone sold! Later on, surprisingly it was seen that people died in that Swine flu fewer than in the seasonal flu. Moreover, most of the deaths were among those who had cancer, Aids, disease of lungs or serious obesity.

To its surprise, the Council of Europe ordered a thorough investigation to find out why the World Health Organization had spread so much scare.

It was seen from the investigation that the bestselling drug for the pandemic was Tamiflu and the manufacturer was Hoffmann-Laroche, a Swiss multinational healthcare company, and the main ingredient of that fill Tamiflu 'Relenza' had been manufactured by GlaxoSmithKline.

The surprise was: some of the panel specialists of WHO, who declared it as a pandemic, were still working at GlaxoSmithKline and Hoffnann-Laroche. In addition, it was also found that scientist and Professor Sir Roy Anderson used to get yearly honorarium of +116,000 (found) from GlaxoSmithKline (GSK). And Nancy J. Cox (virologist), the Head of influenza division of the U.S Government, would get regular financial contributions from GSK and Hoffnann-Laroche for her research works. At that time, Nancy Cox had also been serving as the director of the influenza division at Centers for Disease Control and Prevention (CDC).

Sales of vaccines and drugs -- all done successfully! And the reality is -- Swine flu has never appeared again as a scare.

Some disappointing statements and reactions from the concerned can help us understand how and why the so called Swine flu pandemic was scandalized. The Council of Europe produces a damning report into how a lack of openness around "decision making" has bedeviled planning for pandemics.

Attested by Paul Flynn, MP who prepared a recent report on the flu pandemic for the Council of Europe, a news on Journal of public health (oxford) says, there was a conspiracy theory about nearly everything. So claims that swine flu was a scam come as no surprise. 'This was a pandemic that never really was'.

In conformity with news published on BBC news on 24 June 2010, Newport West MP Paul Flynn says, "Billions wasted over swine flu."

"Billions of pounds in public money were wasted worldwide on buying drugs to combat a swine flu "pandemic that never was", says Paul.

He told BBC Wales' Dragon's Eye the World Health Organization (WHO) made a "terrible mistake" in causing panic.

Flynn said: "They [WHO] frightened the whole world with the possibility that a major plague was on the way."

He added: "The result of that was that the world spent billions and billions of pounds on vaccines and antivirals that will never be used. It is a huge waste of money."

He claimed that the decision by WHO to declare a pandemic had been influenced by pharmaceutical companies.

He said: "The firewall that should exist between the commercial interests, the pharmaceutical bodies, and the scientists has been breached.

Flynn disclosed that the only people who benefited were pharmaceutical companies. They had a huge influence in defining what a pandemic is."

Mr. Flynn said WHO was not being transparent in not explaining who had sat on the emergency committee that had declared H1N1 a pandemic.

Based on the investigation report, a scientist who advised the Government on swine flu was a paid director of a drugs firm making hundreds of millions of pounds from the pandemic.

This is Professor Sir Roy Anderson who sat on the Scientific Advisory Group for Emergencies (Sage), also would hold a £116,000-a-year post on the board of GlaxoSmithKline, the company selling swine flu vaccines and antiviral to the NHS.

After Roy's illegal activity got uncovered, he faced demands to step down amid claims that the jobs were incompatible. 'This was a clear conflict of interest', the concerned said.

How much had gone wasted? Only looking at the U.K, as Mr. Flynn explained," The UK spent £500m on anti-viral drugs that will now never be used." In the U.K it was warned that 65,000 could die as a result of the virus.

The U.K ordered 90 million doses of H1N1 vaccine and only 4.63 million doses were used while all the rest was a big wastage.

The links between the advisors and the companies that make money from vaccines and flu treatments were detailed in a report published online by the British medical journal (BMJ), which investigated the advisors' role in WHO's policy.

It shows that WHO guidance issued in 2004 was authored by three scientists who had previously received payment for other work from Roche, which makes Tamiflu, and GlaxoSmithKline (GSK), manufacturer of Relenza. The key scientists had done paid work for pharmaceutical firms that stood to gain advice they gave to WHO.

The report confirmed that scientists who advised the World Health Organization on its influenza policies and recommendations—including the decision to proclaim the so-called swine flu a "pandemic" had close ties to companies that manufacture vaccines and antiviral medicines like Tamiflu, a fact that WHO did not publicly disclose.

In line with a report, scientists who drew up the key World Health Organization guidelines advising governments to stockpile drugs in the event of a flu pandemic had previously been paid by drug companies which stood to profit.

Randeep Ramesh, social affairs editor says, Trio of scientists who urged stockpiling had previously been paid.

City analysts say that pharmaceutical companies banked more than $7bn (£4.8bn) as governments stockpiled drugs. The issue of transparency has risen to the forefront of public health debate after dramatic predictions last year about a swine flu pandemic did not come true.

This is the picture of a virus pandemic in a world where gambling is also possible. Unfortunately we cannot unanimously depend upon scientists or venerable organizations because they also can get involved in corruption to consume people's money. Such a sad experience of a pandemic certainly urges required justification of the present pandemic that is a matter of pains for every single man of the world.

CHAPTER 2

Coronavirus Myth

Corona or Corona virus has become such a name throughout the globe that we are at a great risk in future. The name as a symbol of scare has got extra weight among viruses. So almost no one is expected to be out of that fear as soon as one will hear the name with its any model reviving. As to me, risk not for its fatality but for fear. There is a saying popularly said in Asia: A burnt child fears fire. That's why we need to travel through Coronavirus junctions to be just known to its large family. It is also to find a way in the face of hundreds and thousands of coronaviruses in future. Though it is a medical term -- the realm of science and research; here we will try to take a view.

As described and defined by Center for Disease control and prevention (CDC),

Coronaviruses are named for the crown-like spikes on their surface. There are four main sub-groupings of coronaviruses, known as alpha, beta, gamma, and delta.

Human coronaviruses were first identified in the mid-1960s. The seven coronaviruses that can infect people are:

Common human coronaviruses

229E (alpha coronavirus)

NL63 (alpha coronavirus)

OC43 (beta coronavirus)

HKU1 (beta coronavirus)

Other human coronaviruses

MERS-CoV (the beta coronavirus that causes Middle East Respiratory Syndrome or MERS)

SARS-CoV (the beta coronavirus that causes severe acute respiratory syndrome or SARS)

SARS-CoV-2 (the novel coronavirus that causes coronavirus disease 2019, or COVID-19)

People around the world commonly get infected with human coronaviruses 229E, NL63, OC43, and HKU1.

Sometimes coronaviruses that infect animals can evolve and make people sick and become a new human coronavirus. Three recent examples of this are 2019-nCoV, SARS-CoV, and MERS-CoV.

So there isn't just one coronavirus. Besides SARS-CoV-2, six others are known to infect humans—four are mild and common, causing a third of colds, while two are rare but severe, causing MERS and the original SARS.

And more is waiting.

The scientists have also identified about 500 other coronaviruses among China's many bat species. "There will be many more—I think it's safe to say tens of thousands," says Peter Daszak of the EcoHealth Alliance, who has led that work. Laboratory experiments show that some of these new viruses could potentially infect humans. SARS-CoV-2 likely came from a bat, too.

SARS-CoV-2 is the virus. COVID-19 is the disease that it causes. The disease arises from a combination of the virus and the person it infects, and the society that person belongs to. Another thing to note is that all types of Coronavirus diseases are mainly respiratory illness followed by some common symptoms like fever dry cough running nose sore throat and tiredness and symptoms become slightly different in respect of different Corona members of Corona family as we have experienced with SARS-CoV-2, SARS or MERS. Just look! All these three names contain the last two letters RS that stand for Respiratory Syndrome meaning trouble in breathing and breathing organs.

Now taking the fact '500 different Corona viruses'! No way to live on Earth! How helpless we are before viruses, especially when the name is Corona! As the first two corona viruses warmed up to rob the human population, the third one has launched a massacre; what will happen when 500 will be infecting one after another, and what about tens of thousands of coronaviruses as said by Scientist Peter Daszak!

Think the only task of the world's population is going to be being chased by Corona viruses and continuously running away to save life under chase. Lockdown shutdown round the year or whenever dragons need more and more money, business is to be multiplied overnight. Think, this way the human population should lose its existence. The planet is set to disappear into space.

Rest assured! Nothing like that will happen. And believe nothing special may be happening now. Probably we are under a big net cast by the fisherman! We need to look to time because time itself unfolds the folded.

CHAPTER 3

Panic for Virus

The Coronavirus myth has made the world almost mad. Situation went such a way that the word 'corona' or the word 'virus' will surely panic us, as most of us are in the dark about virus or virus load in nature and even in our body. As general people we probably don't know the mystery that there are trillions of microbes like virus bacteria fungi inside our body and in our surrounding environment. Our physical system or immune system always outfights the harmful microbes and this way, we can live smoothly. A normal immune system fights disease-causing germs like bacteria, viruses, parasites or fungi and removes them from the body. If we can think of this reality, we won't have to be scared unnecessarily hearing the word virus or even coronavirus too.

We have to be astonished at the quantity of those microbes like bacteria, viruses, parasites or fungi our body are exposed to inside the body and in our surroundings.

As per scientists, the human body is home of trillions of bacteria, viruses, fungi, and other tiny organisms. It has been estimated that there are over 380 trillion viruses inhabiting us, a community collectively known as the human virome.

How many viruses are there in nature?

Curtis Suttle from the University of British Columbia in Vancouver gives a good concept about the amount and activity of viruses:

Viruses outnumber stars by a factor of 10 million. If you lined them all up, that line would be 10 million light years long! To put it on a more conceivable scale, it's been estimated that each day, more than 700 million viruses are deposited from Earth's atmosphere onto every square meter of our planet's surface.

Viruses are like a natural lab seemingly playing around with genetic permutations and combinations.

Viruses also have benefits. Most of the genetic information on Earth probably resides within them, and viruses are important for transferring genes between different species, increasing genetic diversity and ultimately enhancing evolution and the adaptation of various organisms to new environmental challenges.

Some viruses can actually kill bacteria, while others can fight against more dangerous viruses. So like protective bacteria, we have several protective viruses in our body.

How many different viruses are there on planet Earth?

20 years ago Scientist Stephen Morse suggested that there were about one million different types of viruses on Earth.

The results of a new study suggest that at least 320,000 different viruses infect mammals.

What about all the microbes?

It's often said that the bacteria and other microbes in our body outnumber our own cells by about ten to one. That means our average body cell 100 trillion need to be multiplied by 10 to get the number of microbes in a human body, resulting in 1000 trillion. Because of their small size, however, microorganisms make up only about 1 to 3 percent of the body's mass but play a vital role in human health.

Prof Rob Knight California San Diego gives a good concept of this in brief:

No matter how well you wash, nearly every nook and cranny of your body is covered in microscopic creatures.

He told the BBC: "You're more microbe than you are human."

"You're about 43% human if you're counting up all the cells," he says.

Prof Sarkis Mazmanian, a microbiologist from Caltech, says, "What makes us human is, in my opinion, the combination of our own DNA, plus the DNA of our gut microbes."

Skimming through the virus load and overall load of microbes in the body and in nature, we see that we can't go away from those viruses or microbes while trillions are being hosted inside us and are being contacted by unlimited numbers everyday like tiny particles in the environment. As our forefathers could live and we are living plainly through all these, excessive arrangement or unnecessary scare matters next to nothing. Only logical Science matters for us, not Science Fiction to handle virus or Coronavirus.

CHAPTER 4

Naming Strategy

Naming the virus Covid-19 or SARS Cov-2 is such a mysterious case that it would draw your attention. The debate we can find on the naming stage of Covid leads us to looking from some different angles to understand whether there was a logical view behind the name or any intention to mislead the world. Firstly, I will describe the naming stage and debate, secondly naming process and finally we will draw a logical view.

It started out as the "Wuhan virus", with everyone from researchers to news outlets—including those inside China—referring to it as such. Then it was the "Wuhan coronavirus" and "China coronavirus," and subsequently 2019-nCoV. Meanwhile a provisional name was given to coronaviruses of medical significance before a permanent name is decided upon: Novel coronavirus (nCoV)

Finally, on Feb. 11, the World Health Organization (WHO) gave the disease an official name: Covid-19.

In journals like the Lancet and the New England Journal of Medicine, scientists use both "Covid-19" and "SARS-CoV-2" to refer to the disease and virus respectively, but never the WHO's term "Covid-19 virus." But despite the virus having a full name, the

WHO almost never refers to it as SARS-CoV-2. Instead, it uses "the virus responsible for Covid-19" and "Covid-19 virus."

To be clear, Covid-19 refers to the disease. "Co" refers to corona, "vi" to virus, and "d" to disease. The virus that causes the disease is SARS-CoV-2, which was named by the International Committee on Taxonomy of Viruses. The "SARS" part of the name refers to the new coronavirus' genetic link to the virus that caused the 2003 SARS outbreak. So one tests positive for SARS-CoV-2, not Covid-19, as it's the virus and not the disease that does the infecting. The WHO lays out this distinction clearly on its website.

Responding directly to the matter, a group of 12 scientists based in the US, Hong Kong, and mainland China argued that SARS-CoV-2 is in fact an appropriate name for the new coronavirus. The name, they argued, "does not derive from the name of the SARS disease," but refers to its links with the viruses in the SARS viral species. "In other words, viruses in this species can be named SARS regardless of whether or not they cause SARS-like diseases," they wrote. The authors also argue that far from damaging social stability, "keeping SARS in the names of viruses of that species would keep the general public vigilant and prepared to respond quickly in the event of a new viral emergence."

Some have argued that SARS-CoV-2, as a name, can cause confusion. In a letter published in the Lancet, six co-authors from China (including three from the China Center for Disease Control and Prevention) argued that naming the novel coronavirus SARS-CoV-2 is "truly misleading" because it "implies that it causes SARS or similar," especially for those without technical expertise in virology. The authors added that the name SARS-CoV-2 "might have adverse effects on the social stability and economic development" of countries experiencing the epidemic, as "people develop panic at the thought of a re-occurrence of SARS." Instead, they proposed naming the virus human coronavirus 2019, or HCoV-19.

Let's see what WHO thought to name the virus.

We now have a name for the disease and it's 'COVID-19'," WHO chief Tedros Adhanom Ghebreyesus told journalists in the Swiss city of Geneva. The new strain of the coronavirus that causes COVID-19 was named severe acute respiratory syndrome coronavirus 2 (SARS-CoV-2). The WHO writes on its website that it steers clear of SARS-CoV-2 because "using the name SARS can have unintended consequences in terms of creating unnecessary fear for some populations, especially in Asia which was worst affected by the SARS outbreak in 2003." At a press briefing on Feb 13, WHO executive director Michael Ryan noted that SARS-CoV-2 is a technical term for virologists in labs, while Covid-19 is a term for the average person. "We're trying to relate the virus to the world, the experience that people have with the virus... so I don't think there's any inconsistency," he said.

These above lines are a compilation of statements analysis or reasoning from different groups and sectors along with justification by WHO. The purpose is to understand the real picture.

Questions are:

Was there any emergency to give it a new name or to say 'new'?

How logical is the name covid-19 in this respect?

Why had the naming become a matter of debate?

Why is the WHO so reluctant to use the name SARS-CoV-2?

Why did WHO give so much weight to this virus?

In the rest of the writing we will be trying to understand the fact applying common sense and not the bigger Science.

Viruses are generally named based on their genetic structure to facilitate the development of diagnostic tests, vaccines and medicines. But how much should Scientists go on with newer names for a virus or viruses of the same family --- that's really illusive and needs to catch a bigger eye of Science. New naming novel viruses only for medical purposes could be a simple work, but naming according to its origin should be a good work.

SARS and SARS Cov-2 both are Coronavirus, SA for severe acute RS for respiratory syndrome. Cov refers to corona virus and Covid for coronavirus disease. Novel refers to new, so Novel Coronavirus is for new coronavirus.

We find no difference between SARS and SARS Cov because Cov can refer to both; both are of the coronavirus family. And then stands 2 with Cov-2 that should refer to the second sequence of the same or similar previous one. In a word SARS and SARS Cov-2 show no difference except sequential case to be second as we give roll number to a same class students like 1 2 3 under same class identity with some typical differences. In a class giving a serial roll number is a must. But is it also a must to give different roll numbers to significantly same or similar viruses? Many address SARS as original SARS to differentiate it from SARS Cov-2. If SARS is original, SARS Cov-2 is the duplicate copy that is also somewhat clear for its numbering as 2.

Some Scientist say, SARS Cov-2 has direct link to the original SARS, and some were also heard to say that travelling through mutations,SARS Cov-2 has come from that original SARS and somehow managed to show its distinct identity.

Scientists say, virus mutates, meaning that it copies its genome sequence in its progressive term and develops. "It simply means a change in the genome sequence. It doesn't mean that it's necessarily bad for you at all," Scientist Racaniello said. "Plants grow in the spring. Viruses mutate. It's no big deal."

For better understanding of the topic we can skim through one chapter of a book.

W R Fleischmann of the University of Texas Medical Branch at

Galveston wrote in his book Viral Genetics:

Viruses are continuously changing as a result of genetic selection. They undergo subtle genetic changes through mutation and major genetic changes through recombination. Mutation occurs when an error is incorporated in the viral genome. Recombination occurs when co-infecting viruses exchange genetic information, creating a novel virus.

Mutations can produce viruses with new antigenic determinants. The appearance of an antigenically novel virus through mutation is called antigenic drift. Antigenically altered viruses may be able to cause disease in previously resistant or immune hosts.

Recombination involves the exchange of genetic material between two related viruses during coinfection of a host cell.

As I was saying, if SARS Cov-2 is that novel virus or novel coronavirus that is the result of mutations and recombination originating from SARS and if it is an antigenically novel virus that is produced by mutations from original SARS. Perhaps SARS Cov-2 is a cousin or predecessor of SARS. Then how Novel coronavirus should be a name of the virus while it says about new identity only? If SARS Cov-2 is a result of SARS, why WHO should be reluctant to use that name? Another thing is how Covid-19 could be a good name when Covid refers to coronavirus disease as it is a general term that could logically refer to any coronavirus disease of SARS, MERS and anymore? Here, pointing to 19, a year is not enough to mean a separate existence of a virus where a common term is used.

There are findings that this bat virus SARS Cov-2 had 79% identity with SARS-CoV and 50% identity with MERS-CoV.

In this case Scientists' suggestion for the name SARS Cov-2 sounds good from a medical view whereas Covid-19 that WHO craves to use as the official name seems questionable.

WHO said that it does not like the name SARS Cov-2 not to horrify people with their past experience of SARS. What was the condition actually?

When WHO named Covid as Covid-19 on 11 February, Covid-19 had already proved to be more severe than SARS. On 11 Feb only in China 42,708 people had Covid cases and 1017 Chinese died till that day whereas total counting of SARS was 8098 cases and 774 deaths. So will you say that WHO avoided that scientifically suggested name to give people release of fear?

If we think negatively, the name Covid-19 was completely a new name with rising cases and deaths. People had no link of experience to this name as in Covid-19 there is no trace of respiratory syndrome (RS) that they had handled quite successfully, but Covid or the meaning of Covid was new to general people. Using the given name Covid-19 may be ok, but reluctance to use SARS-cov-2 or intention to cover familiar SARS which had already proved to be less severe on the naming day, really makes the question thicker. Unlinking people's experience might show illogical intention when thought of scare is proved baseless. I think due to the newly presented virus cutting all links of existing past experiences, has helped people get over scared that has made the situation bad to worse.

Name matters little, but it matters if you intend to use it for another purpose. We don't have proof or it is quite impossible to prove such intention. But one should accept that a new name could be a good way for new or unknown scare while the severity of the familiar one is far back.

CHAPTER 5

Pandemic Declaration

The word of the year 2020 and even for at least next 100 years, the word which will remain the most memorable is, no doubt, 'Covid-19' or 'Coronavirus' and another word that follows Covid-19 is 'pandemic' that might be the most well-known and most scaring word next to Covid. I should say, this is pandemic not Covid that would be the worst criminal of the 21st century. Pandemic, the horror film for the world's trodden population popularly presented by the lot-makers! Pandemic appears to be a global net cast routinely over this orphan planet. The episode is not pandemic. Rather it is a pandemic declaration. Pandemic appears to be a sovereign demon, a super powerful looter while epidemic is a mere baby. Hence we had better weigh the pandemic and its declaration that has attracted high esteem of fear. Let's explore other two pandemics looking at the platforms they were declared on, with the purpose of examining Covid-19 and its depth of sphere.

SARS or global SARS outbreak is called the first pandemic of 21st century hitting during November 2002 through July 2003. It is a disease, severe acute respiratory syndrome. The whole world got panicked to save their lives on the earth. On the CDC timeline we can find out the day of pandemic declaration for SARS though for its quick dying off, the word 'pandemic' lost its circulation turning to epidemic to most of the people.

March 28: The SARs outbreak is more widespread. CDC begins utilizing pandemic planning for SARS.

Ok, fine, but what was the update of SARS on that day? As per WHO website and SARS chronology, total SARS cases were 1485 followed by 53 deaths till 28 March.

Should we say like 'How ridiculous it was?' and what is the last scene?

According to the World Health Organization (WHO), during November 2002 through July 2003, a total of 8,098 people worldwide became sick with severe acute respiratory syndrome that was accompanied by either pneumonia or respiratory distress syndrome (probable cases), of these, 774 died. By late July 2003, no new cases were being reported, and WHO declared the global outbreak to be over.

And this is the first pandemic of 21s t century, the first terror of the 21st century that appears to be an angry lion for the whole world.

Ok, now let's get on to the next one, Swine Flu, already entitled as a scandal largely disfiguring the glamour of WHO and pointing to greater weakness of the world's fatherly organization. How was the day for Mr. Swine when WHO declared HIM a global pandemic?

As per Timeline June 11, the World Health Organization (WHO) declared a pandemic and raised the worldwide pandemic alert level to phase 6, which means the virus was spreading to other parts of the world.

As of June 11, WHO reported that there have been 28,774 cases of 2009 H1N1 infection and 144 deaths reported by 74 countries.

Look! The then fatality rate 0.5% or one death in each 200

affected a death figure like 144. What happened finally?

18,449 lab-confirmed deaths were reported to WHO while CDC and WHO estimated the death number to be 284,000 (range 151,700–575,400)

CDC says," This differs greatly from typical seasonal influenza epidemics, during which about 70 percent to 90 percent of deaths are estimated to occur in people or 65 years and older."

What a thing! Each dot is to be noted.

But data shows that more people died of seasonal flu the previous year.

As per Journal of public health (oxford):

There is a conspiracy theory about nearly everything. So claims that swine flu was a scam come as no surprise. 'This was a pandemic that never really was' according to Paul Flynn, MP who prepared a recent report on the flu pandemic for the Council of Europe.

Now let's take our final step on to the venerable and Giant Covid-19 pandemic.

Again how was the day for Covid-19 when Covid pandemic was declared?

WHO timeline, 11 March 2020:

Deeply concerned both by the alarming levels of spread and severity, and by the alarming levels of inaction, WHO made the assessment that COVID-19 can be characterized as a pandemic.

And what was the severity and fatality on that day of declaration?

As per WHO on 11 march: There are now more than 118,000 cases in 114 countries, and 4,291 people have lost their lives.

SARS Cov-2 has been addressed as the most aggressive virus with a death rate around 4%. In its progressive term Novel Coronavirus

Cases: 27,561,639 Deaths: 897,989 till 9 September, 2020. Unquestionably both the figures are quite big which have pushed the world to a bitter experience.

In contrast, simple seasonal flu comes to mind.

As a highly contagious respiratory illness approximately 9% of the world's population is affected annually by seasonal flu, with up to 1 billion infections, 3 to 5 million severe cases, and 300,000 to 500,000 deaths each year. According to WHO the death range by seasonal flu is 290,000 to 650,000.

Another thing is that seasonal flu or influenza is not a reportable case in even several states of U.S, let alone other parts of the world while in Covid pandemic something like 'operation search-light' are being run to find out every single case and death of Covid not to underestimate the counting.

Thus far we have some summarized data in hand in context of pandemic or pandemic declaration. We need to know now what features a pandemic has or should have.

As per Bulletin of the World Health Organization 2011:

A pandemic is defined as "an epidemic occurring worldwide, or over a very wide area, crossing international boundaries and usually affecting a large number of people". To say more, a true influenza pandemic occurs when almost simultaneous transmission takes place worldwide. However, seasonal epidemics are not considered pandemics.

And this is the definition of a pandemic!

But from my point of view, there should be more specifications for defining a big thing like pandemics. If we again look at declaration dates of the pandemics for their status, we find the term much controversial that might require reevaluation and reconsideration to block openness to mere intention.

The bottom line is, we are handling unique or separate pandemics with same respiratory illness, nearly same symptoms and same transmission process with slightly up down variations of severity or fatality with virologically unique names, while seasonal influenza is our regular company with similarity in almost everything including crossing borders, simultaneous spreading worldwide and type of the disease.

CHAPTER 6

Misrelated Loss and Damage

Really the planet has already gone under the feet of the killer coronavirus and is going to be crushed too badly. What we have lost and are going to lose due to Novel Coronavirus, are quite impossible to assess because the impact would be found more and more in coming years rather than we have seen till now.

Yet, trying to understand the amount of loss altogether will be a good task. It is also to understand if it was really inevitable or we ourselves wrote down that misfortune on the forehead. We can go through a few of the featured statements to partly understand that loss.

COVID-19 could push 100 million people into extreme poverty, says World Bank. In keeping with the International Labor Organization (ILO) on May 6 2020, 1.6 billion workers are going to be jobless. The figure is jaw-droopingly large: 1,600,000,000. One-point-six billion. That 1.6 billion is the number of people on the margins of the world economy, from migrant workers to those employed in the gig economy, who are in immediate danger of losing their livelihoods. They make up half the world's workforce and it is far from certain that their jobs will reappear even when the crisis is over.

Good news is, the Covid pandemic has come as a fortune for the billionaires. The billionaires have had a huge increase in their wealth in just four months of pandemic. According to a report of Swiss bank USB in October, 2020, the billionaires saw their wealth climb 27% to $10.2 trn from April to July this year with the increased number of billionaires 2,189 from 2,158. And USB said billionaires had done "extremely well" in the Covid crisis. As stated by Business Insider, even in the USA, billionaires saw their net worth $637 billion during Covid pandemic. This is really by the blessings of Coronavirus.

Well, but what is on the other side of the coin? Opposite to that $637 billion, 40 million Americans lost their jobs who filed for unemployment during the pandemic. And what to say about those developing and under developed countries! A recent World Bank report showed 'extreme poverty is set to rise this year for the first time in more than two decades due to the pandemic'.

Additionally, in some reports, suicide rate and divorce rate were foresaid to increase alarmingly.

As reported by the Asian Development Bank (ADB), the global economy could suffer between $5.8 trillion and $8.8 trillion in losses – equivalent to 6.4 percent to 9.7 percent of the global GDP – owing to the coronavirus pandemic. The International Monetary Fund (IMF) says, the global coronavirus pandemic has sparked an economic "crisis like no other," sending world GDP plunging 4.9 percent this year and wiping out $12 trillion over two years.

Disruption to food production and supplies due to COVID-19 could cause more deaths from starvation than the disease itself, as claimed by an Oxfam report published July 9, 2020. The report found that 121 million more people could be "pushed to the brink of starvation this year" as a result of disruption to food production and supplies, diminishing aid as well as mass unemployment. The report estimates that COVID-19 related hunger could cause 12,000 deaths per day: the peak global mortality rate for COVID-19 in April was 10,000 deaths per day.

 In respect of education, COVID-19 already left an adverse impact on education. Almost 24 million children are at risk of not returning to school next year due to the economic fallout of COVID-19, accordant with the United Nation's policy brief on the pandemic's impact on education, released on 04 August, 2020. This huge number of school drop-out might have long lasting disruption in societies.

 How much the pandemic is taking away from the general in assurance of safety is really uncountable. Just to take a hint, as stated in USA Today, New York alone is spending $5B to fight COVID-19 treatment and protection, let alone its up to 50 states or that big world.

All are tax payers' money that would really help some manufactures of medical and protection equipment along with pharmaceutical companies. But, people need to get rid of Covid, so, maybe, nothing to do.

Again, if I am right in saying that misleading panic highly contributed to death from a practical point of view, then who will take that liability? What may be the price of those unexpected deaths beyond the actual disease-related death? In addition, the price of all that agony people were not supposed to bear!

After all, this pandemic is set to the discrimination between the rich and the poor incredibly higher that should be focused to save the fallen. The rich are sharply getting richer; the poor are being promoted to extreme poverty!

And the actual picture of our misfortune is a term to be awaiting.

CHAPTER 7

Severity Concept

Covid-19 is so widely formatted for its severity that, from time to time, concerned authorities utters like "this virus is too aggressive or this is too severe." Is it really for which Cov-2 has managed to top the list in history with an unlimited mine of scare? For a full length realization we need to see the related cases, especially the recent pandemics with their severity context.

First, let's take Covid-19. In its progressive term till 9 September, 2020, Novel Coronavirus Cases: 27,561,639 Deaths: 897,989 with 3 to 4 % mortality rate as per several trusted sources.

SARS had a total of 8,098 cases worldwide, according to the World Health Organization (WHO). Of these, 774 died.

SARS fatality rate stands up to 10% with simple math though many sources state it to range between 6% and 7%.

In terms of Swine flu, only 18,449 lab-confirmed deaths were reported. Suspected cases are stated 700 million to 1.4 billion and out of those infected CDC estimate that 284,000 people died but it ranges 151,700–575,400). That means the actual figure might be between the two. Though H1N1 influenza (Swine flu) tends to cause high morbidity but low mortality rates (1%-4%) according to different sources. But CDC or WHO haven't stated clearly about Swine flu mortality rate, maybe, due to claims of scandalization.

In all the pandemics, most virus-related deaths were estimated to have occurred in people 65 to 90 years of age and mostly who had been undergoing deteriorated health complexities with blood pressure kidney disease heart disease Asthma or trouble in any or more major body organs. Now-a-days we hear about the severity classes so much in the term of Coronavirus, but as if it were new.

Illness severity of Covid 19 by CDC updated on June 30:

Mild to moderate: 81% Severe: 14%

Critical: 5%

In brief 81% of Covid patients suffer mild to moderate and need not go to hospitals. 14% of Covid patients may need to go to hospital or take some treatment. Other 5% get critical who might require ventilation or incentive care. Findings suggest that in case of those 5%, most are found having either age bent complexities or undergoing major organic difficulties like high blood pressure heart disease kidney disease cancer obesity etc.

Again, Covid-19 is too severe! Really? If it is too severe or so dangerous or as aggressive as the concerned say every now and then, why 95% of the infected go out of danger with some or no treatment. This is because a severity is expected to cast a remarkably bad impact on even those who manage to escape from the casualty. What should we say about U.S president Donald Trump when the infected president was discharged from hospital even aging 74 after 3 days of hospitalization with signs of a hale and hearty man? Maybe, some will say, it was medical support that made it. But that will be a reasoning of saving backside beyond the universal trend.

One of the most important things that is counted about severity of Covid-19and that is ' human to human transmission' is so highlighted to be the dreadful cause of its extra severity whereas all the previous pandemic viruses even seasonal influenza show medical proofs to have the same or similar feature of transmission or spreading. To talk about the easy spreading nature of Covid or it is too contagious, we see, even seasonal flu or Swine flu was much more ahead of SARS Cov-2. To talk about high mortality rate of Covid-19, we see that SARS had more than 7% mortality rate with less total infection while Swine flu had mortality rate ranging from 1% to 4%.

In addition Covid-19 has been given a ground to be the most dreadful that assures its finding out possibly most cases and deaths whereas the previous pandemic statistics were partly a matter of probability. Therefore, it should be given time to reconsider and assess the real mark of severity of Covid-19 and to justify the statements floating in the air so that people can read the real story behind the picture.

CHAPTER 8

Transmission Theory

It is the so called issue in respect of Covid-19 that we are now going to look at. Yes, 'Transmission' the biggest mad bell that was rung and rung millions of time that only increased fear and anxiety. This sounds like a transmission philosophy that has never been compared to the recent similar cases or not ever justified under any magnification. It is like the term has been personified as an unmatched cause of Coronavirus infection only for its human to human transmission characteristic.

According to WHO's timeline, WHO mission to China issued a statement saying that there was evidence of human to human transmission. It means that Novel Coronavirus gets transmitted from person to person. To put it in other words, it's contagious and mostly an infected person can easily infect a sound person while both are in close contact.

That solo statement made by WHO worked like octane-offering into the fire of fear people worldwide were rearing up. The statement turned into something like 'transmission theory' in a short while. People had no data presented before them to rest assured by comparing.

Following the unique statement, global media circulated the transmission of coronavirus for people's awareness. And the blind play had begun already. Covid-19 'human to human transmission' had become so big an issue that it immediately resulted in lockdown, first in one state Wuhan which was largely affected, then consecutively the whole world. It is to add that China was safe as it imposed lockdown especially on one state out of big China with no risk to its economy.

The unique term 'human to human transmission' - what a bad news for humans that they can infect others or transmit virus to others. And the infected were being regarded most hated that actually boosted the death toll afterwards. Immediately after huge circulation of transmission philosophy, a declaration of pandemic stepped forward filling the ocean of fear to the brim. Lockdown or shutdown was inaugurated and unanimously celebrated with humans' untold sufferings. 'Human to human transmission' threw human population into artificial graves leaving the planet totally at a standstill.

But many might say, "Why are you going extra miles and giving it a title 'Big talk'? Well, now let's get into the mainstream. Could I ask some questions politely? If 'yes' the questions are like:

1. 'Is human to human transmission' a brand new issue in context of virus?

2. If not new, why did the giant authorities have no interest in saying like ' it is a usual transmission process' in order to relieve people?

3. Why wasn't any relevant data of even flu-like things presented or compared positively by scientists or researchers that would have relaxed people giving extra energy?

4. Why had the concerned authority never said something like: transmission of CO2 is risky but it isn't a new brand of transmis-

sion?

5. Why had not the authorities ever manifested existing flu viruses and the recent pandemics compared to present COV-2 despite nearly full similarities between the diseases?

All these above questions could be answered through compared assessments.

The authorities could have elaborated on Cov-2 transmission compared to other respiratory viruses, but none did. The very truth is that the transmission process of covid-19 is nothing new and nearly the same that our regular player flu or seasonal flu viruses take to get transmitted or the way of spreading. Additionally we will have known how the normal term flu or seasonal flu infection rate and related annual data go and that would be simply stunning.

As per Hopkins medicine website, "Both SARS Cov-2 and flu virus can be spread from person to person through droplets in the air from an infected person coughing, sneezing or talking. Both can be spread by an infected person for several days before their symptoms appear."

And what is to specially note that by this human to human transmission process, every year, up to 1 billion people (approximately 9% of the world population) are infected by seasonal flu worldwide, out of which 290,000 to 650,000 people die meeting the severity.

It is also said that while both the flu and COVID-19 may be transmitted in similar ways there is also a possible difference: COVID-19 might be spread through the airborne route, meaning that tiny droplets remaining in the air could cause disease in others even after the ill person is no longer near.

Look! The last assessment is under dim possibility, never is it sure evidence in all or most cases. Even several researches came out with the confirmation that novel coronavirus does not spread through air as it has got some weight in comparison. So we should say this might or dim possibility is not enough to emphasize on the announcement that cov-2 spreads too far easily & infect people dreadfully compared to other similar viruses or flue, to resist its way of transmission that has made the disease aggressive far enough also.

If we draw a line of comparison between Covid and influenza to understand the spreading issue, seasonal flu every year infects up to one billion, almost 9% of world population, while corona virus has so far infected 0.04 billion. That means around 90 people get the flu per 1000 while 3.36 people have caught Covid per 1000.

This is such a reality that we should have no room to say 'coronavirus is more contagious than seasonal flu virus'. But scare spreads as 'coronavirus is too contagious' as if it had no competitor in the race of transmission. Millions of Covid cases have happened throughout the globe like that in a same congested family one or two members caught this novel virus while others never did in spite of living so close to each other from the asymptomatic stage up to symptomatic infection. Same cases happened amongst people travelling by public transports between gaps of lockdowns especially in south-east Asian and African countries where we viewed streams of people gathering sometimes even during lockdown.

Some cases also caught our eyes like the wife served her middle aged or age bent husband from fever coughing to fully showing symptoms, but the wife was negative. In such tens of cases the wives proved not to have Covid even after undergoing a corona test for suspicion. Some astonishing cases we have eyed or heard every now and then that the wife didn't ever get corona though her husband died of corona infection, who had lived together for several weeks during asymptomatic and symptomatic period of her husband's Covid case. On the contrary, we saw some countries proceed on regular increase in the number of Covid patients while lockdown were strictly imposed and being followed. What should you say about those who caught Covid during their isolated family life for a few weeks and all of a sudden developed symptoms of covid?

All these are really backside questions and we have no way to look to the hollow sky to get the answers.

In keeping with experts, this is actually due to internal physical and environmental conditions of people that resist even entrance of many viruses which is medically confirmed and said to be functional under immunity strength age and so on.

Again the question arises why WHO and CDC did not take responsibility in transmission context to unburden people's load of anxiety and fear with analyzed and compared data presentation and by sufficient reasoning in order to find ways for people instead of too much scare and uncertainty, rather for awareness and strength? Why are all possible negative messages always on the air with not a bit of hope?

It seems that we have no answers at all.

CHAPTER 9

Covid-19 as a Flu

This episode is going to deal with a more technical concept that flue and Covid-19 are different sides of the same coin. One question goes around: "Why can't we say that Covid-19 is just a variation of flue or it is just a cold?" Probably most people will get shocked at this. To settle the thought we need to go forward with essential elements of influenza and Covid-19.

It is not that we are drawing a mere connecting line between flue and covid-19. Rather, we are leading the darkest pandemic also on to a torch light in a dark lane.

Viruses are named and categorized according to their genetic structures. It is convenient for science and research to identify them with different existences. But when disease matters and a wide range of similarities flocks in a junction, it would be easier for people to address them with a known title. For instance, there are hundreds or thousands of bird species, of which all major features are alike. That's why we call them birds in common though scientists need their distinctions in the lab. In question of viruses, people never experience the virus or see it; they only experience the disease. So addressing the disease with its wide range of similarities should be a good and more convenient manner. I think it will not be nonsense if I say 'yes', Covid-19 is a variation of influenza and even all of the coronavirus family and flue groups are just variations of flue.

While scientists and doctors need to make a big bundle of hundreds of factors like genes genome genetics genetic structure genome sequence viral genetics and so on, people are becoming breathless to cope with that ocean and find comfort by looking at what they really experience.

Look at what experts say about influenza.

William Schaffner of Vanderbilt Medical School says, Influenza is a virus that's spread from person to person. It originates, actually among birds and other animals such as pigs. Influenza is a virus that we have in our throats and we transmit to each other when we're in close contact and also when we get the virus on our hands and touch each other and touch our noses and our mouths and that way we can transmit the virus from one person to another.

This statement about influenza virus goes same with that of Covid-19 though it has remained under a veil.

In the Hopkins medicine website we find a good statement of influenza and Covid-19 virus with their coherent features:

Influenza (the flu) and COVID-19, the illness caused by the coronavirus that's led to the current pandemic, are both infectious respiratory illnesses. Although the symptoms of COVID-19 and the flu can look similar, the two illnesses are caused by different viruses.

Lisa Maragakis, senior director of infection prevention at Johns Hopkins explains.

Similarities: COVID-19 and the Flu

Symptoms

Both cause fever, cough, body aches, new fatigue and congestion or runny nose; sometimes vomiting and diarrhea.

Can be mild or severe, even fatal in rare cases.

Can result in pneumonia.

Transmission:

Both can be spread from person to person through droplets in the air from an infected person coughing, sneezing or talking.

Both can be spread by an infected person for several days before their symptoms appear.

From this fuller statement of Lisa Maragakis, in question of the type of disease itself, it is clear that we are getting the same protein from the Indian salmon or jellyfish; or say, the same light from an electric bulb or from a solar light to remove darkness.

But why Covid comes with different severity or higher severity or mortality rate?

Experts say, while many people globally have built up immunity to seasonal flu strains, COVID-19 is a new virus to which no one has immunity. That means more people are susceptible to infection, and some will suffer severe disease.

Just to say about seasonal flu in the U.S. during 2017-2018 flu seasons, estimates indicate that more than 900,000 people were hospitalized and more than 80,000 people died from flu including 185 pediatric deaths. We know all those a little or even not a bit because the scenes were not under camera or on print as in Covid-19.

In this respect, Martin Blaser, an infectious disease expert at Rutgers University in New Jersey, refers to a pandemic and says:

A global pandemic in 1889-1890 that brought more than 1 million deaths globally has been attributed to influenza.

That could mean SARS-CoV-2 becomes a bad flu, or perhaps even just a cold, and that people may be indifferent about getting their COVID-19 vaccine.

It is also on the air about the uncertainty of Corona virus that it mutates too rapidly and is changing itself too unpredictably. Martin Blaser says, thus far, it doesn't appear that SARS-CoV-2 mutates as rapidly as influenza, even though it is an RNA virus.

We see another good example of how similar flue and covid-19 might be, in the eyes of Russian scientists. Virologists at the Moscow State University (MSU) are studying the efficacy of developing a seasonal vaccine to battle both COVID-19 and the flu simultaneously, Professor Olga Karpova, the head of the Virology Department of the Biological Faculty at the MSU, told Sputnik.

I would just like to refer to an article that Kristina Fiore, Director of Enterprise & Investigative Reporting wrote on Med Page Today on September 8, 2020. It goes with the headline -- When COVID-19 Really Is 'Just Another Flu' followed by a sub heading "Imagine a world about SARS-CoV-2 as it is about influenza."

He says, "Each year in the U.S. alone, influenza kills between 12,000 and 60,000 people, and puts some 140,000 to 810,000 people in the hospital, according to the CDC. But there are no calls for social distancing or mask wearing, no shuttering the economy, to prevent transmission."

The statements by the experts and the related information pose two major points ---- why the Medical Science, I can roughly say in this respect, headed by WHO and CDC sticks to notifying that Covid-19 is completely different or unique as if the world had not a bit experience of such type of disease when the disease is just a familiar appearance. Another one is its dreadful severity that was circulated whereas almost all things are the world's common experiences as flu or just as cold, even though in some cases severe or critical leading to pneumonia.

The purpose of this episode is to emphasize on connections between present and past experiences to easily handle the present crisis. This is because man can handle a crisis more heartily with a prior experience of a similar case. And if he hears that he has no previous experience of a completely new situation, he will get frightened. Unfortunately the case of Covid is going like people have been told that they are to face a demon unseen unfamiliar but most powerful, and the demon is in search of anyone around us to swoop down like a hungry tiger.

The messages like this should be enough for any psychological breakdown leaving people in a fearful situation. Another thing is, if one is frightened, you can easily get anything done by one directly or indirectly. This is kind of a field of psychology where psychologists are required to hand on. But if there was no scare, it would not have been possible to lead people to observances like lockdown, social distancing or wearing masks to complete the circle. And I feel like saying, we should owe to that scare and observances. Otherwise, the planet would have been crushed or the human population might have been extinct by that Novel Coronavirus!

As stated by experts, viruses commonly mutate and reach novelty many times in its continuous mutating process. That's why they appear to be more severe after some years with its novel form, as we hear the term 'novel coronavirus'. And you will have heard the famous Covid-19 virus has already had some novel corona viruses or distinct viruses in less than a year! When all are new, who will respond if you call by new? Extremely puzzling the wholesome attempt is to give it an infinite weight throwing the world population into the darkest horror scenario!

CHAPTER 10

Evaluation of Lockdown

After Covid-19 or Coronavirus, the word that has been ghostlier is no doubt 'Lockdown'. Lockdown -- Lockdown of world life indeed! This is a new word coming to have a ground in human memory throughout the 21st century at least. Quite simply we are going to unfold the true picture of Lockdown in a few practical assessments. We will see how absurd and unwise it was to impose lockdown to prevent transmission of Coronavirus. This mandate of WHO to lockdown the world could hardly prove anything but let scare spread wildly and destroy a lot. First, let's get into the real scenes of that lockdown worldwide that appears to be most ridiculous under justification.

To get a summarized global picture of lockdown, we will take a period while the world jumps into strict lockdown. The coronavirus crisis begins by the first of January. It begins to reach its peak in April and May and in many parts of the world later too. For a better comprehension we can take time from 15 March till May 31 because in this period most of the countries of the world experienced harsh lockdown for Coronavirus scare.

On 15 March, 2020, when most countries stepped into lockdown, the worldwide death toll of coronavirus rose past 6,000, with nearly 160,000 infections. By the end of our estimated period till May 31, more than 6.1 million cases of Covid-19 were reported worldwide, including at least 371,000 deaths, according to Johns Hopkins University.

What we see! Amidst full lockdown followed by rigid social distancing and wearing masks in essential movements in the 75 days' period, 160,000 infections rose to 6.1 million infections and 6000 deaths jumped to 371,000 deaths.

So what that so called lockdown did, and what about so called social distancing and colorful masking where regular sharp rises both in infection and death are crystal clear!

Ok, now let's take some countries individually to study the efficiency of so called lockdown.

On 9 March, 2020, the government of Italy under Prime Minister Giuseppe Conte imposed a national quarantine, restricting the movement of the population except for necessity, work, and health circumstances, in response to the growing pandemic of COVID-19 in the country. Duration of Italy lockdown: 9 March 2020 – 18 May 2020 (2 months, 1 week and 2 days)

On March 9 Italy's coronavirus death toll was 463 and the number of confirmed infections in Italy also increased to 9,172.

By the end of the lockdown on May 17, the total number of cases in the country was 225,435, out of which 31,908 people succumbed to the disease.

Look! In 69 days' strict lockdown, death toll rose from 463 to 31,908 and infections from 9,172 to 225,435. Again telling us that lockdown is next to nothing.

Ok, now take the case of the UK.

The lockdown of the UK begins on March 23 and ends on July 4,

2020.

On March 23 the Department of Health and Social Care says, 6,650 people have tested positive for coronavirus across the UK and a total of 336 people have died.

Till 4 July the total coronavirus death toll in the UK stands at 44,131 and the total number of lab-confirmed UK cases is up to 300,000. Here to note that, according to Public Health England on 27 July, total number of lab-confirmed UK cases is

300,111, total number of COVID-19 associated UK deaths 45,759 where after 4 July deaths and infections declined notably. Again we see, in 100 days' sharp lockdown, the death toll of the UK rose from 336 to 44,131 and infections from 6,650 to 300,000. Once again the nude fertility of so called lockdown!

Let's look at another epicenter of Covid 19 for one last time --- Spain.

In Spain lockdown was imposed on 14 March, 2020 with a total of 136 deaths and with a reasonable number of positive cases. By the end of its lockdown on 21 June, as attested by Spanish Health Ministry, total Covid positive cases were 246,272 followed by 28,322 deaths.

Again we see, in Spain's around 100 days' lockdown, death toll jumped from 136 to 28,322 and total positive cases from a few to a big figure 246,272.

What a scene and the planet is that audience! People with zero knowledge of Maths can do the calculation. Lockdown is everywhere -- lock on the door, lock on the face, lock on the leg, even lock on the lot. Virus cleaner is in every nook and corner like shower. However, Coronavirus dances and dances so high! Was it a coincidence or a failure despite honest attempt? What is the basis of the mandate of lockdown that proves a complete failure?

What is the urgency of such an unjustified observance with so much weight? Despite all that inefficiency we find that lockdown is not yet reported to be a failure! Mask is yet to be reported as a garment!

You may say, the situation might have gone even higher if lockdown had not been imposed. But only might have -- you say. What is that higher! Related issues make good sense here. Seasonal influenza with a same or similar transmission model, limits its spread every year. SARS or Swine flu maintained their natural spread limits where no mandates of lockdown like Covid were imposed. They set out on their ways and stopped when they became exhausted. That is the very nature of this type of virus as we see from several past cases.

What did it actually lock --- Our face, our life or our lot? So lockdown! It locked our common sense! It is like a wizard cast a spell, we are all spellbound. We closed the eye, the eye unto real data and have become ever spellbound. A rumor flies in the sky; we all are flying like a jet. It's a horror scene where we are stumbled at the dead of night. Again lockdown! What makes it a sense!

CHAPTER 11

How Effective to Wear a Mask

Novel Coronavirus has changed the faces of the world's population with masks. So how effective is it to wear face masks to prevent coronavirus? Some experts say masks do make sense for certain groups: the ill and health care workers. Once the CDC said, "It is difficult to assess their potential effectiveness." Sometimes WHO was faltering to suggest masks and sometimes it was heard to specially recommend masks for preventing Covid.

But several authoritative sectors are seen to strictly suggest wearing masks and they regard it as the best way to prevent Coronavirus disease.

Experts say that the question whether a mask actually works to prevent transmission of Covid-19 or not, flies in the face of numerous studies and begets controversies to grasp fundamental principles of how viruses behave and how face masks work.

Some say that N95 masks could be effective to an extent for $Co2$ where fabric or homemade masks are a failure beyond question. Many experts say, even the N95 masks used by healthcare workers are pointless in the face of COVID-19. But, why?

As per research, COVID 19 virus particle size is 125 nanometers (0.125 microns); the range is 0.06 microns to .14 microns. The N95 mask filters down to 0.3 microns. In other words, it is asserted that the virus is smaller than the filter on the N95 mask, so the N95 mask doesn't work. Just for comparison: 0.06 microns to .14 microns and 0.30 microns.

Some experts strongly debate the failure of N95 masks and say, the COVID-19 particle is indeed around 0.1 microns in size, but it is always bonded to something larger. The virus attaches to water droplets or aerosols (i.e. really small droplets) that are generated by breathing, talking or coughing. These consist of water, mucus protein and other biological material and are all larger than 1 micron.

"Breathing and talking generate particles around 1 micron in size, which will be collected by N95 respirator filters with very high efficiency," said Lisa Brosseau, a retired professor of environmental and occupational health sciences.

Even If we accept the efficiency N95 for attachment of Cov-2 to droplets or aerosols making it a larger mass together, we cannot settle the debate. Say, a droplet including Covid virus is trapped on the filter of N 95 mask. The droplet immediately evaporates due to air, leaving the virus and other particles. What could simply happen there? Through the breathings, solid or dry viruses could easily enter the body as it is far smaller than the air pass of N95.

 How inefficient a mask could be to protect flue or corona virus? We should have a fantastic and practical experience though it is not a sure science. While the countries went under strict lockdown and people were deliberate on wearing masks, what really comes to? We see something like deaths rose from 300 to 30,000, infections from ground to the sky. Can we give a sure proof by a practical situation where a mask has reduced infections notably? I think that would be a hard task. Perhaps, again we are to go to that "may be" for a backup.

But how much we have spent for that mask, might be some billions. For instance, Etsy is an online marketplace amid hundreds or thousands in the world. It alone helped sell $346 million worth of homemade masks to 4 million people who came to Etsy for masks alone, when hundreds or thousands are lying ahead. Note it, 'homemade mask' that is being said to be pointless by the experts.

If masks are mandatory or highly advisable for Covid, it should have been for seasonal influenza too, where every year up to 650,000 people die with up to a billion infections and many more might remain uncounted due to its unreportable tradition even in some parts of the developed countries, where both the virus spread in similar or same transmission process. But we had never seen before, the world had become that masker!

Finally responding to the debate, most of the people were seen wearing fabric or homemade masks as N95 were in scarcity even for doctors and health care workers. Furthermore, its price was unsuitable for the poor. Why did people cover their faces with normal masks that are considered pointless by the experts? Why didn't the authorities put their clear message about its inactivity where billions of people changed their faces all around all the time? However, if it was useless and unjustified masking this way, it really scared a lot denoting that the situation was too bad.

CHAPTER 12

Hopeless Predictions

Prediction means telling about the future beforehand. A prediction made by a higher authority should have natural value if it is made on baleful facts, wise eyes, unbiased heart to do a good duty in order to guide people logically torching through the dark path. But first of all, that prediction must have a logical value which will complete an estimate. A prediction while unsupported by knowledge facts and wisdom could be nothing but a mere assumption. How logical were the predictions for Coronavirus repeatedly made by the concerned authorities. It's really a question to find an answer for. We can see into a few of those hundreds of Covid predictions to understand the facts.

In the early days of the Covid-19 pandemic, researchers at John Hopkins University predicted that Taiwan would be one of the countries' most affected by the virus. It is located just 130km from China, saw more than 400,000 of its 24 million citizens working there last year, and had almost three million Chinese visitors in 2019.

In a word Taiwan would be an epicenter of Coronavirus. Fine! But what happened really?

After 9 months of Covid progressive period on 9 September, only a total of 495 people were infected by Corona virus out of which only 7 people died and 475 people recovered. A total of 88,748 people had Covid tests that resulted in only 21 positive cases per million. Is it prediction or a rem uttering? Some may say, they imposed strict lockdown and social distancing. Well, most of the countries that became epicenters of Coronavirus, celebrated lockdown shutdown and social distancing as well-planned measures.

 What we had seen! Positive cases were increasing steadily that had numerous proofs apart from eye-view. You may say that Taiwan has managed to stop transmission. But one simple thing is that China and Taiwan had regular entrances of huge numbers of people across the borders and first affected China could easily transmit the virus largely to the people of Taiwan on the eve of lockdown or by those who previously travelled to China or Taiwan before the standstill. But nothing happened like that. What is the mystery there? I will finally unfold that mystery to do the finishing task of the full work.

Let's take another case.On 26 February, 2020 the Independent U.K had a headline of Covid prediction:

Coronavirus could kill half a million Britons and infect 80% of the UK population, government documents indicate Civil servant briefing to ministers on 'reasonable worst case' scenario reveals scale of potential uncontrolled UK outbreak.

Let's step on. The UK population is 67,886,911 and the possible affected 80% would come to 54300000 or 54 million and 500,000 people were projected to die. Well, what is the total by now in the UK?

On 9 September, 2020 total deaths were 41,586, total positive cases 352,560 out of a huge volume of tests.

And about the U.S. it was predicted that 2.2 millions of American may die of Covid-19. But the number is yet below 200k or 0.2 million. By comparison, total world death is around 1 million till now. It is also to say that the United States is always a hot spot of even seasonal flue causing a big death toll every year.

Do you have taste for one more? Ok, Africa, a predicted epicenter of Coronavirus. Let's look into the window. Coronavirus: Africa could be the next epicenter of the coronavirus outbreak. WHO warns on 17 April, 2020.

UN officials also say, it is likely the pandemic will kill at least 300,000 people in Africa and push nearly 30 million into poverty. Ok, now look at the update of Africa Covid stats after 3 and half a month on 29 Jully where the current population is 1.34 billion.

Confirmed cases = 874,036

Active cases = 330,981

Recoveries = 524,557

Number of deaths = 18,498

Note that more than 18,498 deaths should be an everyday death figure due to its large population.

The present situation of Africa doesn't show any turn to go on to that 300,000 predicted as hot water is now coming down worldwide, rates seem to get thinner.

Furthermore, South Asian and Southeast Asian countries were told to be in a very bad situation with Coronavirus infection due to poverty, weak medical support and lower management capacity as was predicted for Africa. Number one South Asian country is India which is ranked as having the second-largest number of coronavirus cases in the world after the USA. Till 9 September, 2020, 4,382,518 people are infected by Coronavirus in India, total death is 74,028. We should know that more than 25,000 people die every day in India due to its large population 1.3 billion. As reported by BBC, 10 million people die in India in a single year. Now, by adding only 3 days' usual deaths of India we get the total Covid death figure so far. I think there is good scope for everyone to understand the mystery.

And now those officials are trying to find so many whimsical reasons to talk about remarkably lower numbers of infections and deaths in South East Asian and South Asian countries.

CHAPTER 13

Panic Contributing to Death

How much stress anxiety or fear can contribute to death and also increase death toll in Corona virus pandemic, is a matter of medical research. But we, who don't have ABC of Science or Psychology, have practical experience of its adverse impact on our body. In keeping with science, that stress is formed when messages containing fear or negative thoughts come to mind. Our subconscious mind cannot primarily differentiate them and take as a truth and apply our system to implement the message. Repetition of that kind of negative messages creates a firm belief strengthening the stress level with some changes in the body. This way the immune system is largely affected and its capability of fighting the body enemies declines.

Our immune system is a very complex set of systems that has to recognize millions of different types of cells and microbes and make a decision about if it's harmful or not. When it recognizes them to be harmful, it kills them and removes them from the body.

The immune system is made up of special organs, cells and chemicals that fight infection (microbes). The main parts of the immune system are: white blood cells, antibodies, the complement system, the lymphatic system, the spleen, the thymus, and the bone marrow.

It is said that the immune system has the primary job of keeping our body healthy and fighting off disease. The immune system cells travel throughout our body and defend it against antigens, such as viruses. It can be compared to a police officer's patrol to protect the body against disease and microbes. Whenever it recognizes any harmful cell or microbe it coordinates an attack and fights them off.

What happens when we are under stress and anxiety? Hundreds of scientific researchers have clear findings that stress hampers normal functions of our immune system.

The Corona virus panic is sweeping the world. When stress, anxiety, worry, overwhelm, depression and isolation are on the highway, they actually reduce the effectiveness of the immune system and make us, and those around us much more susceptible to getting sick. When the immune system is challenged, we are more likely to contract and spread a circulating virus and expose those around us, our communities, and our global population. Here we get affected by a virus more easily when the immunity gets vulnerable.

What was the most unfortunate for the infected at homes and in hospitals is untouchability and carelessness. Doctors, nurses or the dear ones are staying away. Clinical treatment is ok, or kind of thing with no sure medicine. But, is that well-equipped treatment to save life? Modern treatment should be well equipped with not only drugs and surgery, more importantly it also should be equipped with ardent nursing and caressing sympathy that trigger hope of living in the patients. That hope stimulates immunity making a patient prepared for recovery. It is most vital when the term is viral or bacterial infection. But, was there a bit of that care or sympathy?

Additionally the patients were thrown into such a situation that they could not but feel totally unexpected by the world. In such a solid reality, how can you expect that your dry treatment will heal a man of feelings in a crisis? I think it should not be an exaggeration if I say; all was unjustified scare and misleading information that multiplied the death toll of Covid pandemic over the deaths caused by the actual disease.

In this situation we need emotional tools and practices to boost our immune system to fight off the virus as we need physical practices like washing hands and social distancing. Again, unfortunately that kind of positive message is rarely in circulation on the pandemic highway.

This is the immune system that makes our life possible amidst millions of microbes like virus bacteria fungi inside the body and surrounding us. A number of studies in recent years have demonstrated that our own body might be able to fight cancer too, using the immune system to target and kill cancer cells. Some treatments now aim to use the immune system to fight cancer. Moreover, though very rare, some people can even fight off HIV virus with their immune systems, on the word of some research.

These facts make us hopeful of the immune system and assure how capable it is to fight disease or viral infection. The facts tell us why we need to boost the immune system with positive emotional messages to keep it ready. You might say that a message is not itself a chemical so how it can make real changes in the body. If you go some steps forward, it is now a common science factor that a message or thought always affects your body making lots of chemical changes; even some studies show that repeated messages can change and reshape your genetic information guiding your life to a new path.

In this science scenario, when every day's dangerous scenes of Coronavirus worldwide are under camera horrifying us, when people are greatly shocked hearing his or her Corona positive case with no hope to live, when in quarantine isolation or in ventilator, people are being ignored and counting time for death, when dead bodies are neglected by their kith and kin, when family members are leaving their beloved closed doors holding susceptible and leading to death, when no comparisons of data to arouse hope are being shown with positive attitude, when the solid reality is remaining under a big veil, when a gorgeously dressed up rumor run by the selfish and the corrupted is dominating the world, how badly the immune system is being swept expediting the death procession!

CHAPTER 14

In order to assess how much severe Covid-19 is, which aspect is mostly used, is the total death number along with death rate. In this phase we are going to look at the heavy death toll caused by covid-19. But, why? The purpose is to try to understand the actual death number of covid-19 exploring some chances and evidence of over counting the number. This is also because the good number of Covid deaths might represent wrong severity making people panicked and misleading them to manage the pandemic. Some trusted statements we have come across, tickle the possibility of the over counting the death number and under some evidence it is vivid that it is not the actual number we have seen so far.

By the time this book is in progress, we see the total death number of Covid-19 is 885,021 as on September 6, 2020. It is quite a big figure for people to get alarmed actually. But let's see how a big complexity lies in making this figure and how different authorities or concerned sectors address that issue.

According to the website of public health England under the heading "Behind the headlines: Counting COVID-19 deaths" Posted on 12 August 2020, in context of defining a COVID-19 death, it states, "Although it might seem straightforward, counting the number of people who have died from COVID-19 related illness is complex."

The World Health Organization (WHO) also recognizes this complexity and states that:

"A COVID-19 death is defined for surveillance purposes as a death resulting from a clinically compatible illness in a probable or confirmed COVID-19 case.

However, it is only an approximation of the number of people who die from COVID-19."

NBC News takes a look at how some of the world's health authorities have tried, and often failed, to keep track of those who have died in the pandemic. It says, "Official coronavirus death tolls are only an estimate, and that is a problem."

On the word of Johns Hopkins University, "while the official global death toll stands at more than 126,000 that number represents a mere estimate. Only countries with extensive testing can confirm their mortalities and, even in those with the necessary medical technologies. The simple act of counting the dead reflects the chaos that COVID-19 has wrought."

The National Institute of Health reports that in Italy, people who die in hospitals with the coronavirus are deemed to be dying of the coronavirus. On re-evaluation by the National Institute of Health, only 12 percent of death certificates have shown a direct causality from coronavirus."

Again, a study conducted by the Superior Health Institute and National Statistics Institute reported to the National COVID-19 Surveillance System on 25 May "COVID-19 was the direct cause of death for 89 percent of patients who died with a positive test for the virus in Italy. It adds that the direct cause of death for the remaining 11 percent of cases has been attributed to several other health conditions."

Another study of England examined 41,598 deaths in confirmed cases of COVID-19 reporting up to 3 August 2020 and found that: 88% of deaths occurred within 28 days of a positive COVID-19 test and 96% occurred within 60 days.

But Public health England in a post on 12 August 2020 states that a death in someone who has tested positive becomes progressively less likely to be directly due to COVID-19 as time passes and more likely to be due to another cause. Mark the words, counting within 60 days might go so chaotic and uncertain to count or certify Covid deaths while 28 days is a medical standard.

I need to go further miles to clarify on that.

While Public Health England address the issue saying "counting the number of people who have died from COVID-19 related illness is complex", we can't rest assured on the accuracy of counting Covid deaths.

While the World Health Organization (WHO) recognizes the complexity, uses 'probable or confirmed' and states that it is only an approximation of the number of people who die from COVID-19, we have a big room to say the figure is progressively unjustified or inaccurate.

When NBC news says that: Official coronavirus death tolls are only an estimate, and that is a problem, we see some counting with closed eyes.

When Johns Hopkins University says: that number represents a mere estimate, none would be eager to accept that so-called death number of Covid as accurate.

Ok, now let's look at Italy. If we take up the statistics that only

12% of Italians' deaths were certified with Covid, what about the other 78% that has already made the world figure fatty? This is questionable as this percentage was not cut out of that total Covid deaths previously added.

Similarly, if we take another study conducted by the Health Institute and National Statistics Institute on Italian death toll and believe it where 89% were assured to die of corona, again question arises: what about another 11% that had no relation to Covid but was first counted to make the total?

So what are the breaches here? Don't you feel like asking some questions? I feel like thinking more but find no answer. It looks like all are busy whole heartedly to maximize the Covid death number and no way let it go underestimated. Why are we all so careful about counting the heads even under approximation and mere estimate leaving not a hair, while struggle for keeping line of accuracy should have been the only target? Here again shall I have to leave you with no answer. Yet I can say if statistics start to talk with their mouths, 'information terrorism' might be a new title to address such cases.

CHAPTER 15

Deaths in Perspective

We are now capped with a huge death toll from covid-19 so far and everyday a big number is being counted adding to the huge toll. No one in the world could be happy with his or her own death news in advance and even none with mental fitness can help being sad hearing any death, let alone that huge death toll of Novel Coronavirus. Everyone should try his best to save every life at every moment that is unquestionable. The World has already had a bitter experience of 885,021 deaths of cov-2 worldwide as per news today on Sep 6, 2020 while this page is under writing. No play! Really corona has cut a good figure and it's really a sad memory for the human population. All should mourn over around a million graves.

But over this gloomy reality, let's try to see the death toll in perspective.

Actually we have nothing to do while we have to embrace 153,424 deaths per day, 6,392 deaths per hour, 4,679,452 deaths per month and 56,000,000 deaths per year worldwide due to several reasons like disease accident homicide and tobacco use. We can't anyway stop this procession of deaths.

To categorize that huge death number, let's look at some major casualty sections.

According to the Center for Disease Control & Prevention, 290,000 - 650,000 die of seasonal flu worldwide every year.

Almost six 6,000,000 people die from tobacco use and 2,500,000 from harmful use of alcohol each year worldwide, the World Health Organization (WHO) reports.

WHO reports that 17.9 million people die each year worldwide from heart disease, an estimated 31% of all deaths worldwide. According to WHO, Cancer is the second leading cause of death globally, and is responsible for an estimated 9.6 million deaths in 2018.

As stated by Reuters, the report explains that tobacco is expected to kill 7.5 million people worldwide by 2020, accounting for 10 percent of all deaths.

As mentioned by WHO, close to 800,000 people die due to suicide every year, which is one person every 40 seconds. It also says, there are indications that for each adult who died by suicide there may have been more than 20 others attempting suicide.

As stated in another report of the World Health Organization, road traffic injuries caused an estimated 1.35 million deaths worldwide in the year 2016. That is, one person is killed every 25 seconds. As stated by the Global Burden of Disease study, just over 400,000 (405,000) people died from homicide in 2017.

The real scenario is that, covid-19 total death number compared to above statistics is reaching a single million despite all those arrangements. The number is nearly as much as that of yearly suicide and far fewer than of road accidents. Tobacco kills people around seven times as much as of Covid-19, alcohol around three times, heart disease nearly twenty times and cancer approximately ten times.

To get a clear picture, tobacco vs covid 7 : 1, alcohol vs covid 3 : 1, CVD vs covid 20 : 1, cancer vs covid 10 : 1

Furthermore, we see that Covid-19 total death is closely equal to the world's only 6 days' death count. In comparison to seasonal flu Covid goes some miles ahead: 885,000 compared to 290,000 - 650,000. If we draw another plain picture by comparing Covid death 885,000 to yearly suicidal death 800,000 as suicide has no pandemic current around us, we see, Covid should not have been so big a talk of the time though awareness and measures could be a way.

In the U.S alone Covid-19 has swooped too badly taking 192,933 lives as per data on September 7, 2020 while many times more are being added to the total death number of U.S. According to CDC, more than 700,000 people die in hospitals each year in the US.

In 2017 in the U.S there were 2,813,503 total deaths. That means 863.8 deaths per 100,000 people. Heart disease added 647,457deaths, cancer: 599,108 deaths, Accidents: 169,936 deaths, Chronic lower respiratory diseases: 160,201 deaths, Stroke: 146,383 deaths, Alzheimer's disease: 121,404 deaths.

Compared to above death statistics of the U.S, Covid toll is 192,933, far less than death toll by heart disease or cancer and quite close to the number put by accidents and some other common diseases individually as mentioned above.

I wonder, as the authorities have been doing so much for coronavirus, how much more they should have done for those killer diseases and life taking problems.

China and India have also gained the fame of notable death toll by Covid-19 while each of the country sees around 25,000 deaths overall everyday due to their large populations.

Notice, all those death statistics put above are not to minimize the importance of 885,000 valuable lives dropped off by the claw of coronavirus. Rather, those comparisons make us much optimistic with consideration and solid reasons. From this discussion, I think we can clearly shout that Covid-19 can never loot our big hope for staying alive, nor it should leave us totally pessimistic while most of the windows are open to breathe. Death is as natural as everyday's sunrise and sunset.

In a sense it is as common as dropping off leaves and blooming in spring. A good thinker will never add huge panic and illogical fancies to a havoc maximizing the loss. Rather, he will stay on his feet and try best to do whatever he can, to minimize the loss. If we hear of a demon in a dark jungle, we should focus on the size, strength and severity of the demon looking back to our tested experiences, applying justified logic and related past data coupled with future probabilities, and then do best to curb the demon.

No good comes when we start hue and cry or rush to and fro in panic. As people of modern age, don't we have to have freedom of mind to differentiate between rumor and reality? We shall have to consider evidence and data along with environment and logic to justify any big cry like Covid Pandemic. We may accept all unjustified things but this nature is alien to the growth of civilization. And this very trait has made our today's civilization possible.

CHAPTER 16

Panic Not Awareness

Scare in the Covid pandemic has become a matter of big concern, a matter of revised thinking. By the blessings of the media -- mass media print media electronic media print media global media, whatever names you give, have played the key role and took the control of the pandemic. More than 70% of adults turn to the internet to learn about health and healthcare, a team of researchers in Canada said. In fact, our life is largely guided by the media in this internet age. It's a matter of hope as long as it can go with good.

To talk about the media, they collect news and present them. In the Covid pandemic, they played the key role to send news across the countries and keep people updated of the pandemic. It is true that people were benefited by the necessary information and unfortunately got affected by fear that was mixed in the news.

If we want to justify the role of the media and think that it somehow casts a bad impact spreading fear of pandemic, we need to justify the news sources that delivered or provided the news.

It is like a chain -- global media, country media, and local media. Global media is a body consisting of some powerful platforms which is followed by other media while you can also say; global media is a total combination. However, definition matters little here. This global platform with a pandemic which is a scientific and medical factor, is widely dominated by the concerned policy makers along with scientists and doctors.

Actually if we step more inside, those policy makers of the giant platforms who have gained global leadership, played the key role. Some statements of trusted sources upheld the negative role of social media in the Covid pandemic. Social media that has no accountability as other medias due to decentralization.

"Social media rules. That's bad in a pandemic," says CNN on May 15, 2020. It states that popular social media posts are filled with inaccuracies about science and they could damage public health during this coronavirus pandemic, according to the authors of two separate studies.

One study found that more than one in four of the most popular YouTube videos about the novel coronavirus contained misinformation. Another found that vaccine skeptics were winning the battle for Facebook engagement.

Journal of medical internet research finds that social media has played a key role in spreading anxiety about Covid pandemic.

But wasn't there any authority to take measures to control that mislead of social media?

As I was saying about global media, but are how those news delivered by the policy makers or any faulty news? Not that, but they transmitted the news only highlighting how harmful Coronavirus is, how much weight this virus has got, how many people it may infect and kill, how helpless the world is under the virus and so on.

The authorities mostly neither compared this virus to the similar past viruses in a positive way nor did compare the normality. For example, they never highlighted the fact that Covid-19 has 81% cases mild to moderate who need not even go to hospitals; another 14 % patients need to go to hospital and recover with some treatment. They never focused on this 95% and said this disease is 95% safe and has no threat for lives. This 95% of statistics were just a mere part of data lying on the sheet or scroll.

Reversely by the media, other 5% severe cases were specialized that are mostly for those age bent or having major organic disorders, where out of this 5, 3-4 may lose lives. They were rarely found assuring people not to be panicked. This harsh reality negatively made a strong ground of scare from personal level to state level, continental to global.

Maybe, some will say, "this is your responsibility to reason the data to assure yourself. Then how it could be reasonable when they are on the gear and accelerator for the pandemic world!

Now, coming to the matter of 'awareness'. Awareness always goes with sympathy and assurance. Pandemic awareness should be encouraging by assuring the safety rate and heartening to fight for the real severity rate with proper measures.

But reversely, what policy makers kept doing! They predicted thousands of times and say like:

How many people may be infected by Cov-2?

How many people may die.(For example: In Financial Express, published on Sep 5, 2020, "The global Covid-19 death toll could reach 2.8 million by January 1, about 1.9 million more from now until the end of the year.")

The whole world is under the Corona trap.

Your life is at full risk if you catch it.

Covid19 is too severe, too aggressive.

The whole world is struggling against an unseen enemy.

Still no way found to save life from Covid.

Look! How big those words are to push people into the ocean of uncertainty! How big those lines are to break down human immunity! Those words together could present a picture like the world population is sinking and struggling to breathe in a big sea finding none or nothing for help. Even most ridiculously many say, "Not fear but awareness is the victory", when the predictions have already closed all doors of hope.

And finally something like 'vaccine is the only way to live on the earth.'

Psychology is, if you just merely walk through the long safe path without interpreting that that long path is safe but keep shouting on the short breach, logically people will keep listening to you and only focus on that breach. They will certainly be tensed up for that problem. They are prone to forgetting that long safe road that you did not uphold. They care about your shout because they trust and follow you. They believe that you are for them. They also believe that you always think for their welfare.

The policy makers, the Scientists, the doctors and the researchers -- all those are in the place of people's belief. Probably they should have been more comprehensive rather than doing mere home tasks. They could have thought that they themselves were the victims to find a way for people. They should have played a logical role without being dominated or being ample followers-- logic that global statistics and data give after unbiased analysis.

Again the role of the media! If we believe that scare was spread intentionally, the media was the only way. Maybe, they themselves did not spread fear or no reason to spread fear. Rather, the media was used to circulate news containing intentional scare. It is the media that has made every global day a day for us staying anywhere anytime. It is media that we cost almost nothing for, to keep updated. And the media is the only leader that can clear up all mysteries of the Coronavirus or pandemic to help the whole human population.

CHAPTER 17

Vaccine Uncertainity

The covid-19 pandemic or corona virus scare finally finds its way to the vaccine, the only way to live on the earth by fighting off the coronavirus. But, is it urgent for people in common? How much efficient will the vaccine be to protect us? These are questions from many experts and lots of controversies are there around it. In terms of efficiency of coronavirus vaccines which are under trial, what scientists are saying, is so frustrating.

How effective are the vaccines going to be? How much efficacy a vaccine should have?

Gathering all the information till today about the efficiency of the coronavirus vaccine, we can say, it may be only 50% effective.

Dr. Anthony Fauci, chief of the National Institute of Health and Infectious Disease says, "We don't know yet what the efficacy might be. We don't know if it will be 50% or 60%," Fauci said during a Brown University event in August.

In other words, scientist L.J. Tan, chief strategist of the nonprofit Immunization Action Coalition explains, "If you vaccinate 100 people, 50 people will not get disease." In other words, you have 50% chance of catching the virus even after taking the vaccine.

According to a study published July 15 in the American Journal of Preventive Medicine, coronavirus vaccine's effectiveness may have to be higher than 70% or even 80% to give some relief in maintaining social distancing. By comparison, the measles vaccine has an efficacy of 95%-98%, and the flu vaccine is 20%-60%.

Note, with that level of 20%-60% efficiency of the flu vaccine, up to 650,000 people die every year in the world. Furthermore, many scientists have doubts about how effective the vaccines will be for the aged and for the obese. Scientists say, it is yet to see how much the vaccines can trigger immune response in those persons. This is because, as we hear, biotech corporations are reluctant to disclose enough information about their individual research for the patent and pricing purpose of the vaccines. We also hear that scientists are not at liberty to disclose their updated findings relating to Covid as they are confined to the biotech corporations or pharmaceutical companies. As a result, the way of running information is hampered.

However, getting back to the point, the aged and the obese, both the levels are worst victims of corona virus disease when vaccines may not be blessings for them. The interesting thing is that vaccines might be unnecessary for 81% with mild to moderate infection who don't have to go to doctors and another 14% who recover with simple treatment. If we make an imaginary calculation, 4,762 people per million are infected by corona virus. Then, do the rest of the people 995,238 per million, really any need of vaccine? This is only for understanding the urgency of vaccine before or after infection. But, then who are projected to vaccination?

Besides, some experts tend to say," If there could be different vaccines for different countries due to immunity and environment!"

Even WHO also expresses that all corona virus vaccines may not work fully to give protection or all vaccines may not work equally. That means different vaccines of Covid 19 may give different levels of protection while all may be around 50% effective.

Again this 50% efficiency goes uncertain, according to some experts. The effectiveness of a vaccine is measured on the basis of trials. The difference between efficacy and effectiveness is that the former applies when vaccination is given under controlled circumstances, like a clinical trial, and the latter is under "real-world" conditions. Typically, a vaccine's effectiveness tends to be lower than its efficacy.

All these uncertainties about corona virus vaccine give insufficient hope of protecting the disease to a considerably effective level. These also pose questions about urgency or necessity of corona virus vaccine in the world when all these are yards of the long way and when similar diseases are left uncared with tens of yearly deaths.

Marilyn J. Roossinck of Pennsylvania State University says, the mysterious disappearance of the first SARS virus, and why we need a vaccine for the current one but didn't for the other.

Accordingly some have questioned why a vaccine is so urgently needed now to stop the spread of the current coronavirus when a vaccine was never developed for SARS. Some people have already questioned why the current coronavirus has brought the world to standstill while a previous deadly coronavirus, SARS, did not.

Moreover some scientists predict that SARS cov-2 will be weak at a stage and might disappear like SARS. British cancer doctor Prof Karol Sikora recently claimed that the current COVID-19 pandemic would "burn itself out".

More traditionally in respiratory viruses, we see that they gets weaker and go just as seasonal, as A(H1N1) virus that caused the pandemic in 2009 subsequently replaced the seasonal influenza.

While there is no sure vaccine for A(H1N1) that takes huge toll every year multiplying the deaths to a horrible total, while no vaccine for the father SARS with his child already in limelight, only urgent issue is vaccine for Covid 19 or corona virus, the terrorist of 21st century!

Should the authorities look back to the past memories to settle the vaccine issue? In this Covid vaccine reality, governments will may be revise the facts to decide whether to spend hard-earned public money to stockpile million doses of vaccine at the cost of billions of dollars.

But should we seek for lasting solution?

Did the world take lessons from the history? Did the scientists explore the past pandemics? What have they learnt?

To look back to the past pandemics, Spanish flu pandemic of 1918–1919, mother of all pandemics caused millions of deaths but ended within two years with no vaccine invented yet. The 1889–1890 flu pandemic, also known as the "Asiatic flu" or "Russian flu", was a deadly pandemic that killed about 1 million people worldwide. This also had no sure vaccine but ended in around two years. Swine flu pandemic has been entitled as "Scandal" and considered as a conspiracy theory. What should we learn here and what is simple?

All flu and corona viruses cause respiratory diseases with similar symptoms but may be more or less severe when they emerge as novel ones. The number and category of respiratory viruses are really horrible with future possibilities as scientists find. All the pandemic viruses weakened their claw in around two years, then disappeared or merged as seasonal with less severity in contrast. This is because people develop hard immunity against those viruses through infection and the viruses become weaker in the combats.

The lesson we can take for Covid-19 is that it would be gradually weaker in approximately two years and we can see clear signs of its decline. What about vaccine for Covid-19? All are under way, some are on trial. After trial more time is required for production. After production it will take months and years for vaccinating a large number of people throughout the world to build mass immunity. Look at the time -- the virus is slowing down and enough time required till immunization. Does it really make sense for people to take the vaccine even though the virus is so aggressive? Won't there be misuse of the money of the Governments or their taxpayers' like Swine flu case as we saw in Britain?

How will you support that the vaccine is the way of saving yourself when it is around 50% effective or how will you emphasize its urgency when the virus is going down?

Some are heard to say that it may rise anytime and can hit badly. I should say, depending on that 'may' is opposite to what we can learn from the history. Waves are under its natural gesture as fire goes up before extinction. I think that hope of vaccinating billions of people would be a hard task or most people would be reluctant to take it, though so many people may take it due to fear. Some billion doses of vaccines are going to be sold for some trillion dollars; money will go from the down onto the upper. That might be a big blow in the business world. But is it going to be good news for people -- is a question lying yet.

I wish I could suggest a way. There is really an effective way in my sense. May be, you all would laugh at it. But I believe it might be a great and lasting solution. What is that? It is nothing but the immunity that can be a way out accompanied by scientific measures and medical treatment. It is the immunity that makes our life possible in the sea of viruses; it is the immunity to which all those respiratory viruses have bowed down. Make your all efforts centering the immunity worldwide. Support your immune system with changes like diet, exercise, stress management and lifestyle.

Support your immune system by caring physical and mental health. Nurture your immunity taking all possible measures. That should be an expedition worldwide by those powerful authorities. This way 100% of Covid infections will turn into those 81% and 14% making nearly all safe. And good news is when the world go change its lifestyle, manage stress, have proper dieting, take regular exercise, stops smoking and taking alcohol, can you imagine What will happen?

As a result, immunity will go wild and sharp decrease of death toll in all the top killers like heart tobacco, CVD, alcohol, cancer will come by product. It will require time but no doubt, it will be a blessing for the world beyond all that mess.

CHAPTER 18

Reality of Covid-19

We have seen how terribly the pandemic paralyzed the world making the most horrible scenario. The world is still dedicated to finding a way against the unseen enemy. Unfortunately I have to say, this planet would have rarely had any problem by the amount of study research awareness dedication and activity that it has invested in chasing the Novel Coronavirus. And millions of encyclopedias would be required to write what has been done with people or people have had to receive worldwide --- to write people's sad stories in the name of Coronavirus.

Inhumanity has crossed all limits in the plea of horrifying social distancing. Tens of incidents and stories put up our naked image of humanity and civilization when we neglected the dying people in suspicion of corona, though in most cases they were corona negative tested after deaths. Our inner brutality and higher grade of selfishness came out when we left sick people to die uncared untreated and untouched in old age homes in many countries. I do not know how to estimate the cost of that kind of helplessness or cruelty. I do not know if some of those who have knowledge, power or authority would be awakened by the heart-rending scenes to save the orphan world.

When I am going to conclude my debate, to our utter surprise, so mysteriously the Covid pandemic is showing clear signs of gradually dying off or the power of Covid is declining after some months of its debut! Yet the horrific world is anxiously awaiting a coronavirus vaccine. Bad news is scientists are undergoing a lot of troubles to make the vaccine and again there are questions about future efficiency of vaccines due to mutations of the virus.

The world is still spell bound and overwhelmed with fear though they have seen that not so much happened as was predicted. Not that happened we have seen throughout here comparing statistics. All the related statistics have shown that the pandemic was given unjustified weight; it was swelled up with scare covering all reasonable data and statistics that should have been shown to assure the fallen people. It was filled up with whimsical predictions or only predicting the negative sides like death and infection. Even when the pandemic itself might be a question, a totally unjustified scare is seen to have spread.

To give a summarized concept, the corona virus disease itself has caused far less havoc than that barren lockdown & scare or we can say, rumor did. The damage caused by the disease itself can never be compared to that the world has lost and is destined to lose in near future. If one says, it is a big fight, we should say, a good strategy of winning a fight must be to win at a minimum loss. If you tolerate maximum loss for a win, breaking down your backbone into pieces and relaxing in relics of loss everywhere, that so-called win will go in vain and remain unsupported.

Probably we should say why we did not handle the virus in the way we handle flu virus every year, with some additional measures (after all, it is a new guest) which is nearly the same as corona except the genetic identity-- same type of disease, same transmission, in a sense nearly the same severity. We hear no calls for wearing masks, no calls for lockdown or social distancing where millions of lives have been lost in recent years in total. We could have maintained everything possible without that fruitless lockdown saving the backbone. Certainly that would have been a good choice or one of the best alternatives.

It may seem that I am breaking code of conduct in the civil world. But I believe I am not talking about what does not really exist. I am trying to show you a small hole in a large ship that no one has seen or everyone left unseen. History may find that breach for some trillion dollars. You may say, "Shut up", like all are closing eyes. But when you are about to strangulate me, I should at least have the right to utter.

Ok, you may not have any interest in what I have seen. But what if there is an unrealistic circle encompassing our lot? Don't we need to pray to our superiors for breaking that vicious circle? People may be indifferent to talk like me for three reasons: Firstly, if they don't understand the facts or have no intention; secondly, if they love to stay in blind illusion and finally, if they are not bad guys like me. But, what solution? When we do not back up the truth getting callous, the truth itself explodes and causes lots of havoc. I wonder if it is going to be a permanent deal to reoccur any time at the sweet will. And that might require immunization for future protection; but not only with a vaccine but also with a good will. If really that exists, should we submit to exploitations, even with our generations exposed to that?

In the pandemic world, irrelevant out-show has covered the real picture of the virus leading people to a rough mixture of rumor and reality, and it is so tough for people to differentiate how much it is real and how much it is a rumor. A conscious man or even a person with common sense might see that the corona virus has been dramatized by a huge crown of rumor and unjustified scare, only when he stands on the statistics and realizes the trends.

 In the context of Covid-19, if we hope to get right answers to the questions that arise in the mind or the questions put forth in our discussions, scientists will need more research and above all, need to restore the chastity; the policy makers will need to be plainly honest and to work for people, not just for their own sake.

All the reasoning and rationality that we have had so far in the book poses a final question -- Was lockdown a must or should be a must in the future probable pandemics? I cannot give you a sure proof nor have the right to do that. Rather, it is a crucial message that emphasizes on settling down -- whether or not, should have or should not, must or never.

We have so far noticed that there were baseless lockdowns, exaggeration of severity, dubious naming formula, inaccurate death number, unscary death toll in perspective and overweight of the term. All these pose questions about the essentiality of the pandemic, absurd celebration of infertile lockdown.

So, is it possible that Covid-19 pandemic is a scandal like the Swine flu pandemic scandal?

If we dive into real data and analyze them with an unbiased mind, chances are much higher because related world data and statistics seem not to support it to that extent the world has really experienced.

If some wise readers carry the message and some experts take heart to interpret the facts, this call will surely have the ground to help the world. Otherwise, it will vanish like a dew drop in the morning sun. Hopes are that the billions of people who suffered badly might try to justify the call and test the message, not just honoring big guns' statements as blind followers.

If you want to settle the issue, you just need to apply common sense; no huge study or research is important as I have no ABC of Science or Viral Genetics. This is because it is a kind of trick usually applied by gamblers taking advantage of a crisis. If someone with authoritative power names it a Global scandal that might sound amazing. But you or me, none is the authority.

So we can't certainly say that it was a scandal or home task. I could only say, the roots of possible scandal might be very deep. This might be a case like we cannot see the bottom of the sea only by looking at its surface waves. If it was a scandal, it was really a bad psychology game. I just held the issue under suspicion, analyzed and reasoned the data and statistics; consecutively have found it suspect. Only the concerned authority can ensure under proper investigation whether it was a scandal like Swine flu or not.

Finally, scientists are the guardians of the civilization. They should take action again for mankind shaking off all influences or greed. They are no doubt superior and the maker of this glossy world. But they should bear in mind that any chance of their moral degradation will spoil the balance of civilization. It has become a moral question, not a matter of knowledge right now before the world. They shall have to put a big hand and prevent Science from turning to willful fiction. Libraries guide life, but if a library covers life, it will merely puzzle people.

Scientists are expected to do something so that the virus issue does not make a mess misleading the world life now and in future. I hope experts will look at the issue to clarify if such pandemics or declaring pandemics with a mess or infertile lockdown to kick down the world is inconvenient and unnecessary or it is all right. Certainly it would be a big welfare move for the whole world population in the near and further future.

Also, the concerned authorities must make concerted effort to save people from that foggy lockdown myth and fearful social distancing. They must think that general people are the worst losers and also they should see if there are any hidden beneficiaries of the pandemics.

Otherwise, the so-called pandemic session will never end and keep the world squeezing. Now lockdown is established, mask is for scare, distancing is like for ghosts -- all these are trump cards for the selfish and the exploiters. So future pandemics could go so easy to grasp the throat of the planet. Perhaps, the world will be preparing for the next routine pandemic of another Novel Coronavirus with a polished name and different strategy. So what? Again, like gentlemen we are ready to accept as our bad luck!

Let's get the last scene of the pandemic. The word population is the audience of a film. It is the most dreadful horror movie. Everyone in the audience is feeling like a fish out of water. They are so into the scene that they could think nothing out there. No one could ever shout for help as if the ghost would swoop down tracing his or her presence there. They are almost dead by the deadliest demon. When the lights are on, they find that they are ok nearly as usual.

The screen is now plain white. Some have said 'goodbye' to the earth as usual or derailed by panic, but badly uncared and untouched. When the audience gets back home, they find they have already lost their jobs. They find that their homes are relics of fear. They are burning inside the cover. Many are predicted to die unfed. Many more are destined to extreme poverty. To mitigate the situation big guns are collecting funds, but they do not know what is in store for them. Amid all these they are messaged to spend some more for immunization to protect against the demon they had seen in the movie.

They are also being told that vaccines may not work fully with 50--50 chances; yet vaccines may save their life. They could imagine that the demon may come any time and many more demons are likely to swoop down in future. They are in the fancy of "may be" as they had been in "may be". When so called predictions fail, they are told how much might have happened.

They do not know the truth, nor have cravings to know. They know what they have been told and how things were told. The demon of scare is now pushing them into a feeling of uncertainty where many struggle and a few can live.

And this is a suggested movie in the coronavirus world.